"*The Goddess in You is more than a simple cycle tracking resource; it is the tool that has been missing from the pro-period generation's toolkit. The empowered embodiment of our daughters depends upon not only their menstrual education, but the connection to their sacred nature. With the goddess archetype as their foundation our daughters are given the blueprint to grow into powerful wise women.*"

AMY BAMMEL WILDING – author of *Maiden's Journey: A Coming-of-Age Circle for Mothers & Daughters*

"*A simple and beautiful invitation to help girls build a relationship with their menstrual cycle. We highly recommend this book for all young menstruating women.*"

ALEXANDRA POPE & SJANIE HUGO WURLITZER – co-authors of *Wild Power*

"*A beautiful resource... Both psychologically sophisticated and delightfully simple to use, I warmly recommend this book to girls, parents and schools.*"

JANE BENNETT – author of *A Blessing Not a Curse*

"*The Goddess in You offers a powerful, creative, and developmentally appropriate path for girls to get to know and love their bodies, menstrual cycles and selves even deeper.*"

MELIA KEETON DIGBY – author of *The Heroines Club:*

Title

THE GODDESS IN YOU

Text Patrícia Lemos
Illustrations Ana Afonso
ISBN 978-1-910559-352
Design and illustrations anafonso.com
Copyright © 2017 Patrícia Lemos and Ana Afonso

English version published by Womancraft Publishing, 2017
www.womancraftpublishing.com

A percentage of Womancraft Publishing profits are invested back into the environment
reforesting the tropics (via TreeSisters) and forward into the community: providing books
for girls in developing countries, and affordable libraries for red tents and women's groups
around the world.

Womancraft Publishing is committed to sharing powerful new women's voices,
through a collaborative publishing process. We are proud to midwife this work,
however the story, the experiences and the words are the author's alone.

This book is dedicated
to the Antónias in our lives

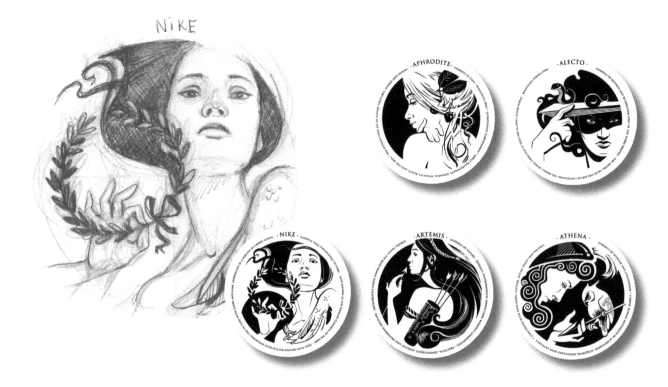

Greek goddesses

In this calendar, you'll find thirteen goddesses to guide you through this journey of discovering your body and yourself.

You will be able to choose a goddess for each menstrual cycle. Each goddess has her own interests, skills and motivations, just like every girl. Each one has virtues and vices. All together, the goddesses represent the full range of human qualities. You may well feel connected to more than one of them, or different ones at different times.

You can also choose goddesses to inspire you to develop new skills and abilities or to give you some extra

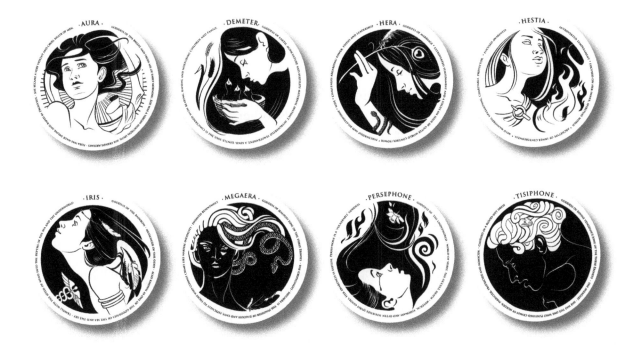

motivation when you are in a specific phase of your life.

You can cut out the goddesses if you would like, and organize or display them, according to your own needs and present challenges.

For instance, let's imagine you're going on holiday to somewhere in the middle of nature. During that menstrual cycle, you might want to summon Artemis – an adventurer herself, as the goddess of nature and animals – to help you get the most out of those days. Or, if you need to study hard, Athena can walk you through that cycle, inspiring you to create a space of wisdom in your life.

Meet the goddesses

All of the goddesses featured in this book come from Greek mythology. You may already have come across some of them, whilst others may be new to you. We hope that they will inspire you as you become better acquainted with them. We offer you just a brief introduction to each goddess, but if you are drawn to find out more you can explore their myths in greater detail in books and online.

 Aphrodite • Goddess of love. She represents passion, selfless devotion, beauty in all things and the arts. Her symbols are a seashell and a golden apple.

 Artemis • Goddess of nature, animals, environmental protection and women's communities. She represents the regenerative power of the Earth in all living things. She's practical, adventurous, athletic and prefers solitude. Her symbols are the bow and the deer. Sister to Athena and Aphrodite.

 Megaera • Goddess of jealousy. One of the three Erinyes or "Furies"– her name means "the grudge keeper". Moved by endless resentment, she stalks those who commit crimes of marital infidelity.

 Persephone • Goddess of the underworld, death and rebirth. She lives in-between worlds and is the reason for the four seasons. Winter settles in when she's away from her mother, Demeter. Her symbols are the narcissus and the pomegranate.

 Hera • Goddess of marriage and childbirth and also the Queen of the gods. Protects partnerships and relationships. Wife to Zeus. She is jealous and vengeful of his lovers. Her symbols are the sceptre and the peacock. Sister to Hestia and Demeter.

 Tisiphone • Goddess of divine vengeance. One of the three Erinyes or "Furies"– her name means "the avenger". She punished crimes of murder and is usually clothed in a dress wet with blood.

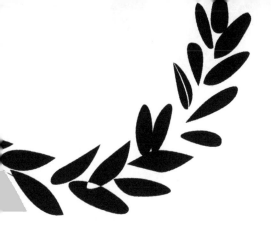

 Iris • Goddess of the rainbow. She is the messenger to the Gods and travels with the speed of the wind.
She represents flexibility and being able to let go of limiting beliefs.
Her symbol is the rainbow.

 Demeter • Goddess of agriculture and fertility. She represents the maternal instinct.
She makes spring happen every time she reunites with her daughter, Persephone.
Her symbol is a sheaf of wheat.

 Hestia • Goddess of hearth and home. Never married, herself, she protects the household and families. Focused on her inner world, she's welcoming and pacifying.
Her symbol is a sacred flame.

 Alecto • Goddess of revenge and retribution. One of the three Erinyes or "Furies" – her name means "the unresting one". Punishes those who commit moral crimes. Alecto and her sisters, Megaera and Tisiphone, have wings, and serpents in their hair.

 Nike • Winged goddess of victory. She flew over battlefields rewarding the victors with glory and fame. She represents inner strength and the will to overcome difficulties. Her symbol is a laurel wreath.

 Aura • Goddess of the breeze and fresh air. She's one of the virgin-huntresses. Once a carefree spirit, she was punished for comparing herself to Artemis and went mad. Her symbol is a billowing veil.

 Atena • Goddess of wisdom and war. Motivated by her keen intellect and concerned with education, culture and politics. Her symbols are the owl and the olive tree.

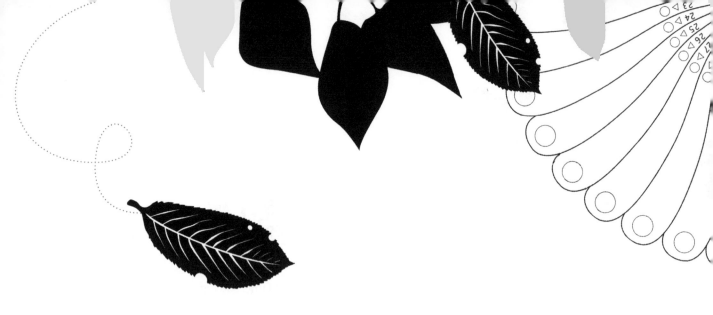

The Menstrual Cycle

Getting your first period is an important milestone in your life: it means you are well on your way to becoming the woman you will be.

Every girl is different. Some will start menstruating when they're nine years old, others won't get their first period until they're fifteen or older. Some will have a regular menstrual cycle from the time they get their first period, whilst others will have just a little light spotting and then wait several months until menstruation settles into a regular rhythm.

Healthy cycles can vary from 25 to 35 days but it can take a while to get into this rhythm as your body is still maturing.

It all starts in your head, with your pituitary gland pulsing a hormone that will signal to your ovaries to release a tiny egg, no bigger than a pin head. These phases are called pre-ovulation and ovulation and go on unseen inside you.

During this time, your uterus (also known as your womb) starts building up a fleecy blood bed (called the

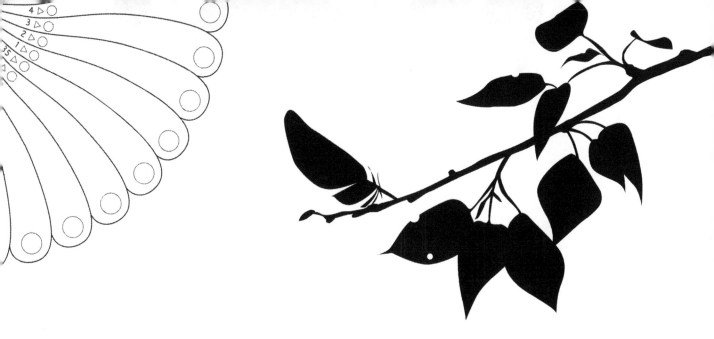

endometrium) deep in your lower belly. This is where the egg will nest if it comes to be fertilized by the sperm from a man, when (and if) you decide to have a baby.

Approximately two weeks after ovulation, the endometrium is shed, and that's when you get your menstrual blood. Your blood marks the end of a cycle, and at the same time, the beginning of another, because it all starts again. So, more than just preparing us to be mothers, the menstrual cycle, with its wonderful internal dance, helps us learn about the cycles of life. About beginnings and endings. Just like day and night, the moon phases, the tides and the cycle of life itself.

The most important thing is for you to remember that the menstrual cycle, periods and body changes are normal events in a healthy woman's life and should be celebrated.

During your first menstrual years, your body will be trying to find its own rhythm but you can help it adjust with some basic self-care activities that will also allow you to live your menstrual cycles in a healthy and comfortable way.

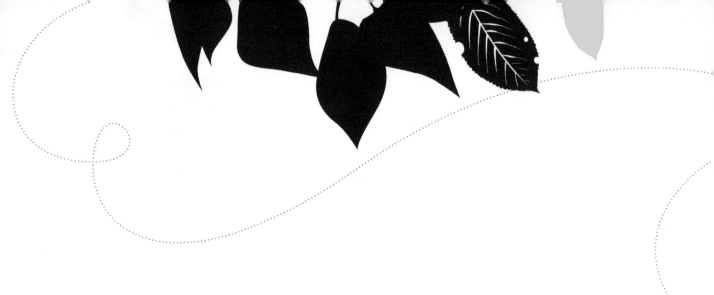

Remember the four seasons – spring, summer, fall, winter? Let's use their initials (**SSFW**) to help you recall these four basic self-care tips to help you to look after your body throughout your menstrual cycle:

Sleep – make sure you mimic the day's natural cycle (wake up with the sun, go to sleep with the stars); this will help you rest enough, regulate your cycles and help you connect with the rhythm of the universe.

Satisfaction – make to sure to do something every day that makes you happy. Create space in your life to do things for yourself (and for others) that help you to feel accomplished and satisfied. This might be sports, crafts, reading a book, cooking... or whatever it is that you like to do. Remember that you can always count on a goddess to help you with this.

Food – don't skip meals! Be sure to make healthy, nourishing as well as delicious food choices. If you suffer from menstrual cramps you might want to

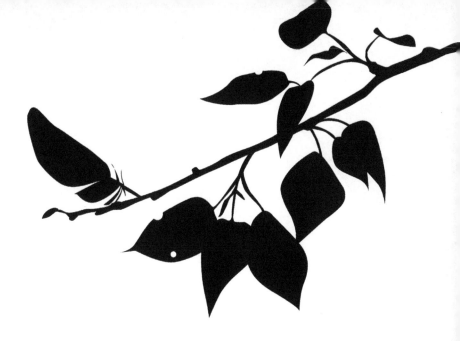

reduce your intake of both dairy products and sugary foods during the two weeks before your period.

Water – make sure you are well hydrated so that your whole body is working at its best. During your menstruation this also helps your uterus contract effortlessly, avoiding menstrual cramps and pain.

If you find yourself worrying about your body changes, you might want to reach out for help and talk about it with your mum, sister, friends, a teacher or someone you can trust.

In ancient times, in the time of the goddesses, long before periods gained a bad reputation, women used to gather when they were menstruating to help and support each other, sharing experiences and stories about their lives. You can do the same with a couple of friends, to find out more about each others emotions throughout your cycles and help each other if you're having trouble dealing with some aspects of your life. That's what goddesses do.

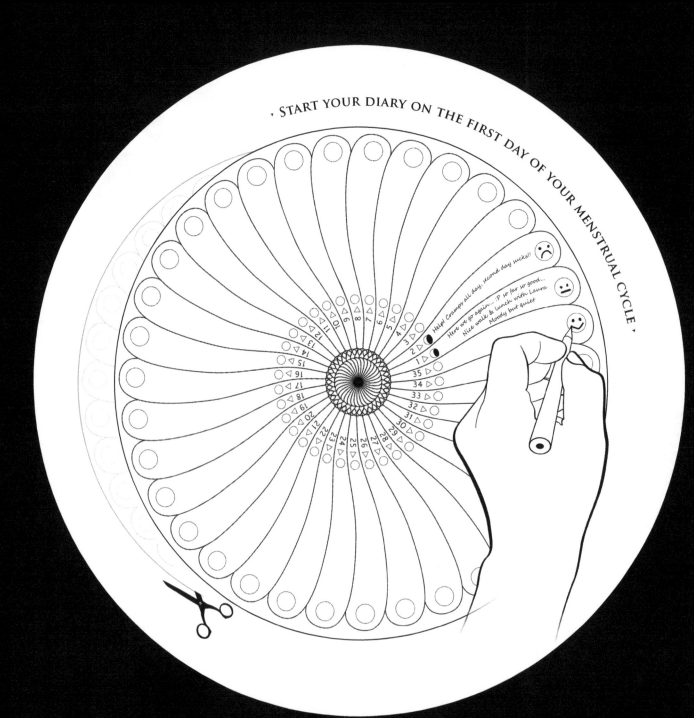

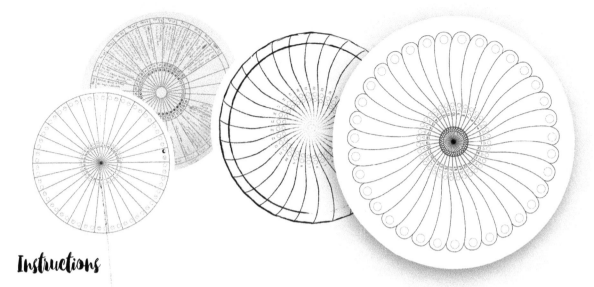

Instructions

1. Each cycle mandala in your calendar has 35 days but your own menstrual cycles may vary from this as well as from one cycle to another, without it being a problem. Remember that your body is still adjusting...

2. The first day of a menstrual cycle (day 1) is always the one in which you start bleeding and when you begin filling in a new menstrual circle.
Each segment in your cycle mandala corresponds to a day of your cycle and it offers free space for you to write about it, include information about the phase of the moon and even an emoticon that will help you describe how your day went.

3. Take time to look back over previous month's mandalas. The information you gather will help you to understand your menstrual cycles and how they make an impact on your daily life.

4. The more time goes by and the more cycle mandalas you fill in, the easier it will be for you to discover patterns within yourself. Soon, you'll find out that there are times when you feel energetic or creative, and others when others when you feel angry or sad; times when you'll want to be surrounded by friends, and others when you feel like just being by yourself, enjoying the silence and doing nothing. This is the cycle within you.

5. You can colour your goddesses using coloured pencils or crayons and cut them out, if you want to.

Ready? Here we go!

Choose your goddess

APHRODITE

"I WAS BROUGHT INTO THE WORLD ON THE FOAM OF A WAVE. I TRANSFORM THE WORLD THROUGH LOVE AND BEAUTY, BUT MY VANITY CAN CAUSE DISCORD."

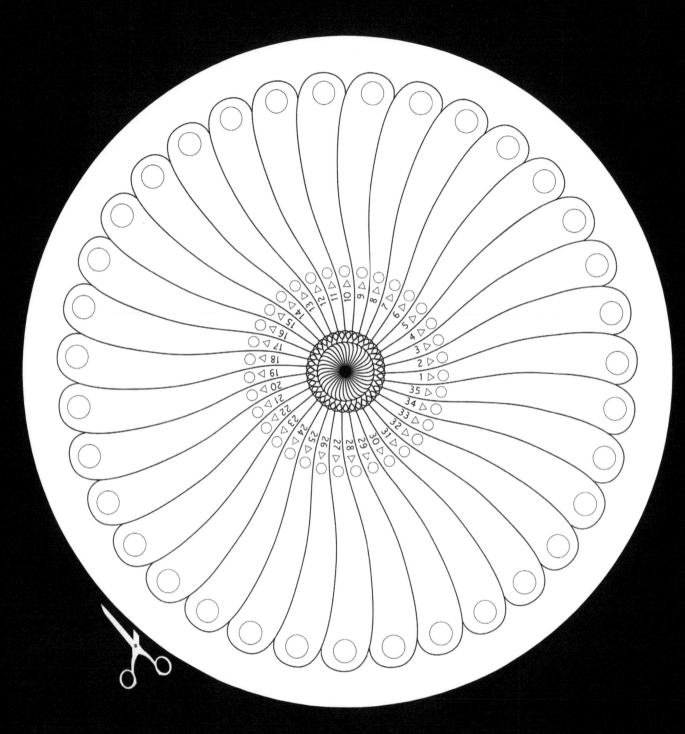

ALECTO

"INJUSTICE MAKES ME ANGRY. I TRACK DOWN THOSE WHO HAVE COMMITTED WRONGS AND PUNISH THEM."

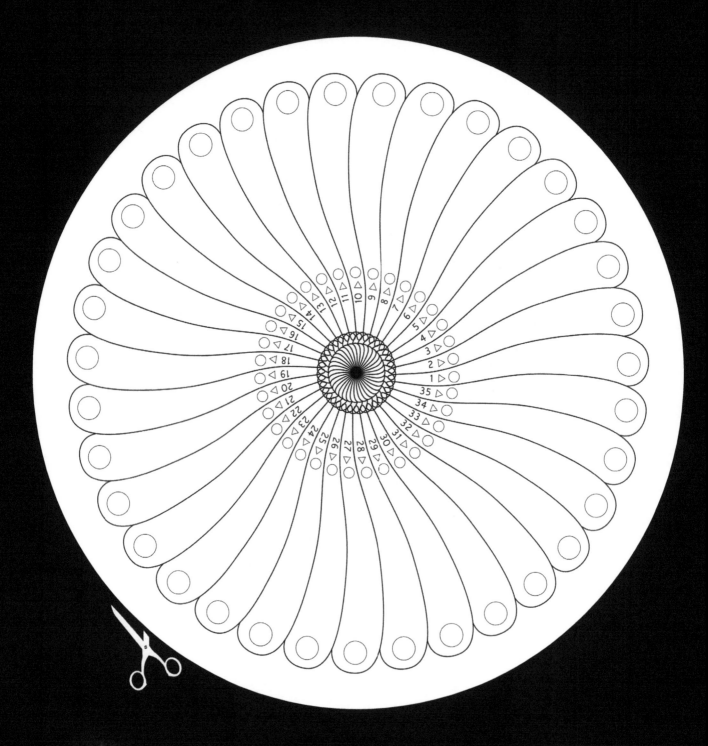

· ARTEMIS ·

"I CONNECT WITH THE EARTH AND RESPECT MOTHER NATURE ABOVE ALL THINGS. I AM SKILLED WITH MY HANDS. A LONELY HUNTER, I AM GUIDED BY THE MOON"

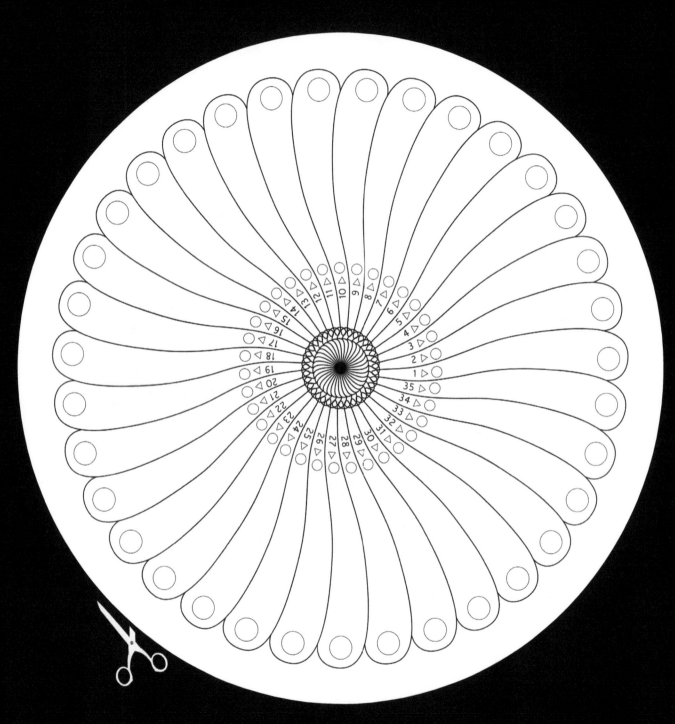

· ATHENA ·

"I AM SELF-MOTIVATED AND DRIVEN BY MY INTELLECT. I STAND AGAINST INJUSTICE AND THE SUFFERING OF OTHERS."

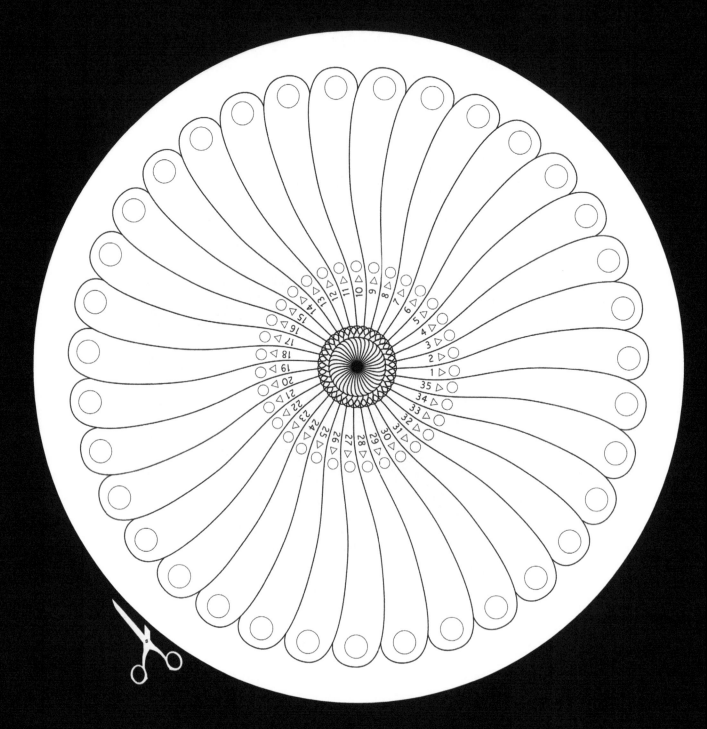

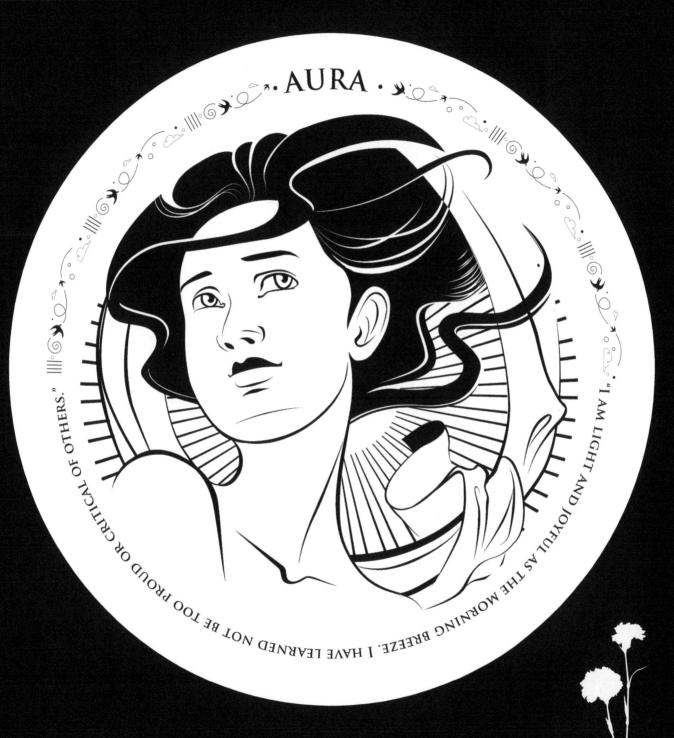

· AURA ·

"I AM LIGHT AND JOYFUL AS THE MORNING BREEZE. I HAVE LEARNED NOT TO BE TOO PROUD OR CRITICAL OF OTHERS."

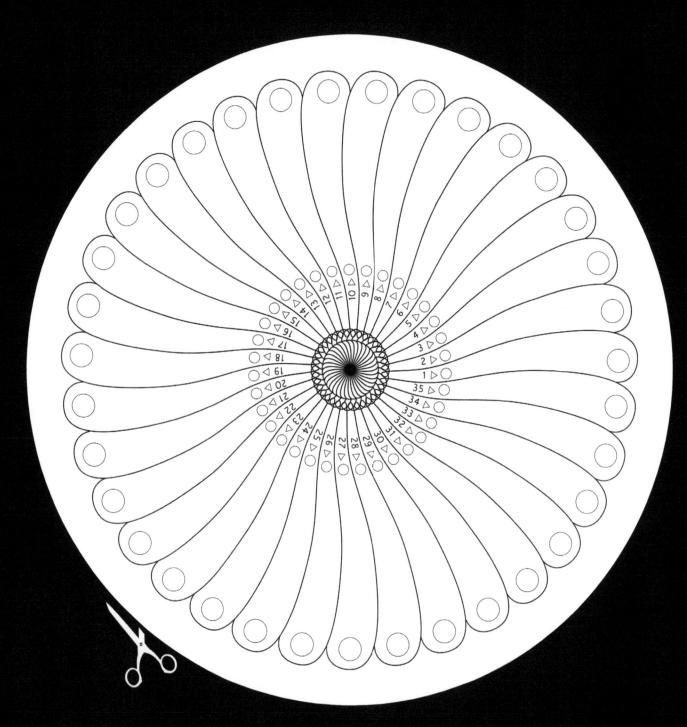

DEMETER

"I HOLD THE WISDOM OF THE CYCLES OF NATURE AND THE SEASONS, I TEACH THE JOY AND LOSS OF FAMILY RELATIONSHIPS."

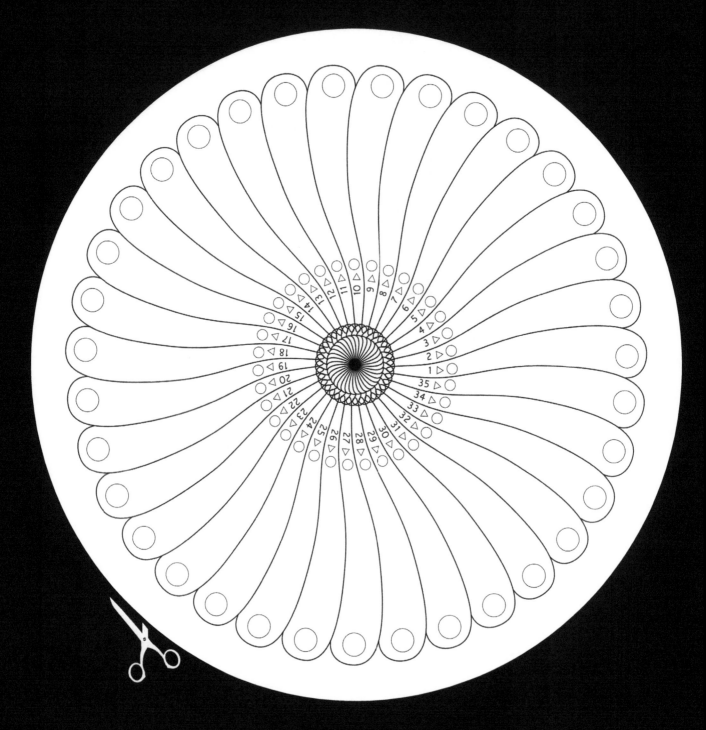

HERA

"I AM A QUEEN. I BELIEVE IN PARTNERSHIP AND BLESS ALL LOVING RELATIONSHIPS AND THE BIRTH OF NEW CHILDREN. BUT WATCH OUT, I CAN BE JEALOUS."

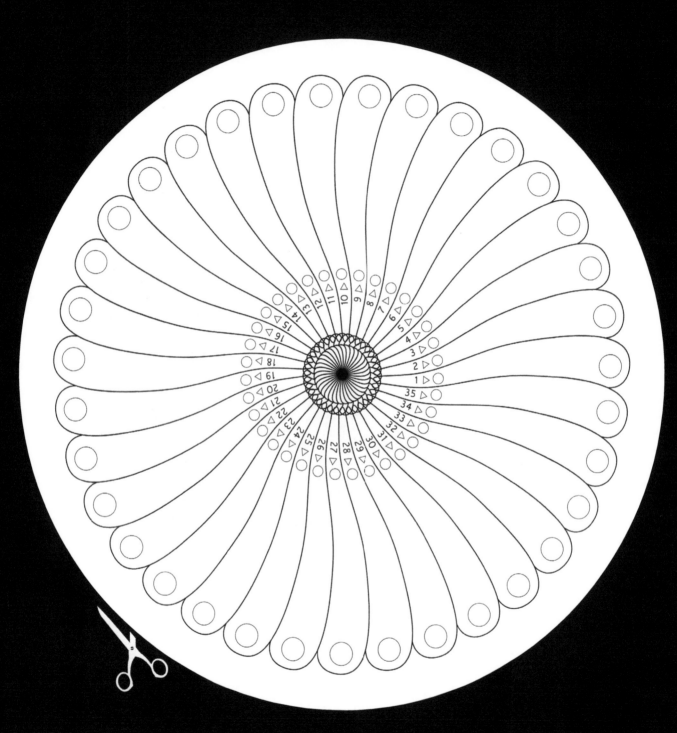

· HESTIA ·

"I KEEP AWAY FROM DRAMA AND STAY FOCUSED ON MY INNER STRENGTHS. I DO NOT NEED A MAN TO COMPLETE ME. I AM HAPPY IN MY OWN COMPANY."

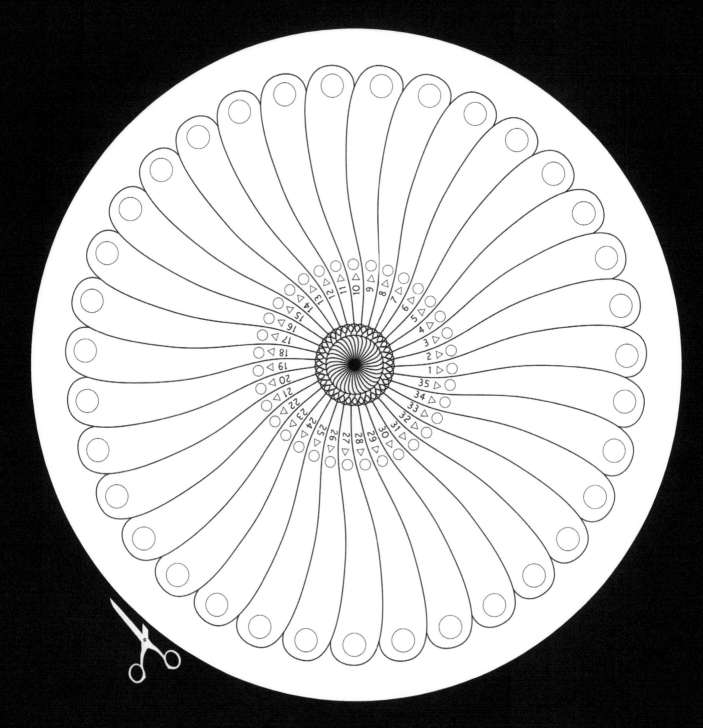

· IRIS ·

"I SEE LIFE IN BEAUTIFUL COLOURS. I SHAPE MYSELF TO THE ENVIRONMENT AND CIRCUMSTANCES AROUND ME, AND AM ABLE TO BALANCE OPPOSING FORCES WITH GRACE."

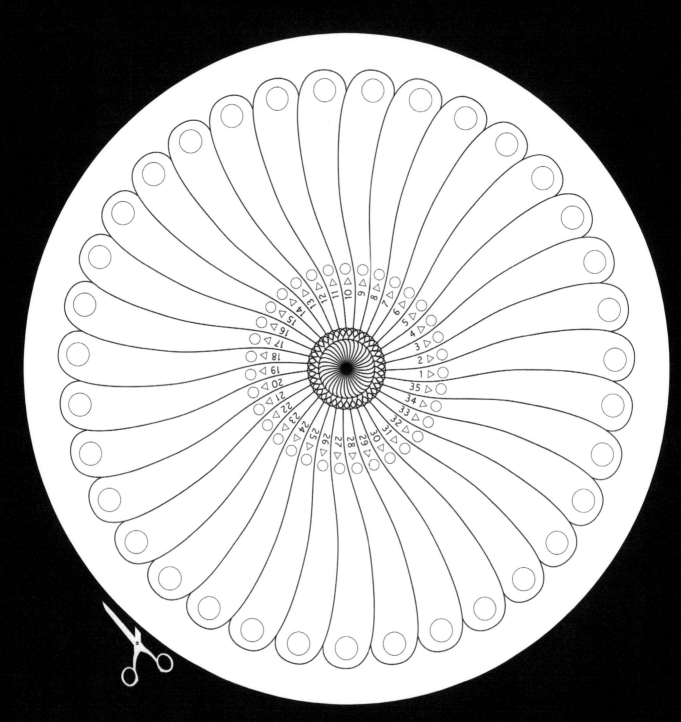

MEGAERA

"I ALWAYS FIGHT FOR THE TRUTH AND I HAVE AN EXCELLENT MEMORY, I REMIND THE UNFAITHFUL OF THEIR FAULTS."

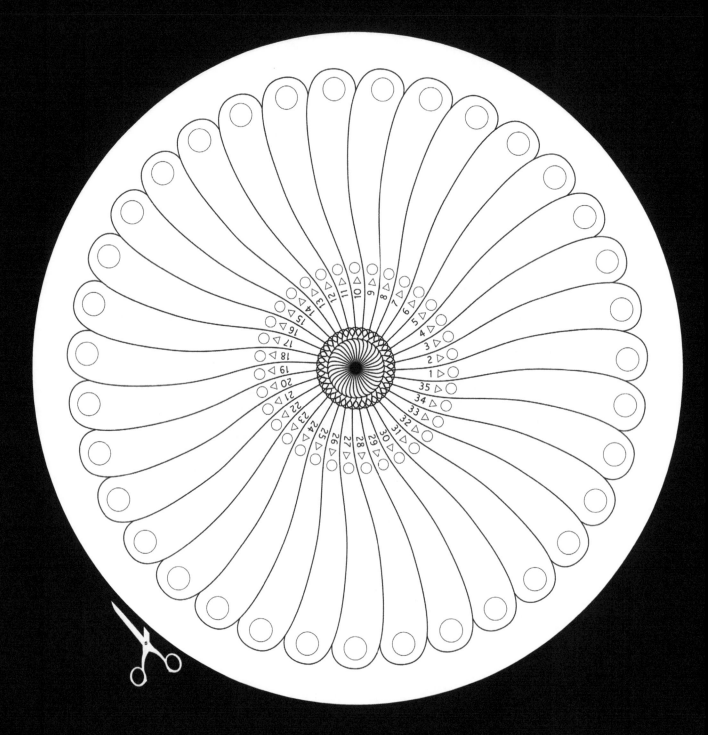

NIKE

"I COME TO WIN. I RESPECT MY OPPONENTS AND STAND FOR PEACEFUL AND FAIR COMPETITION. I THRIVE IN SUCCESS."

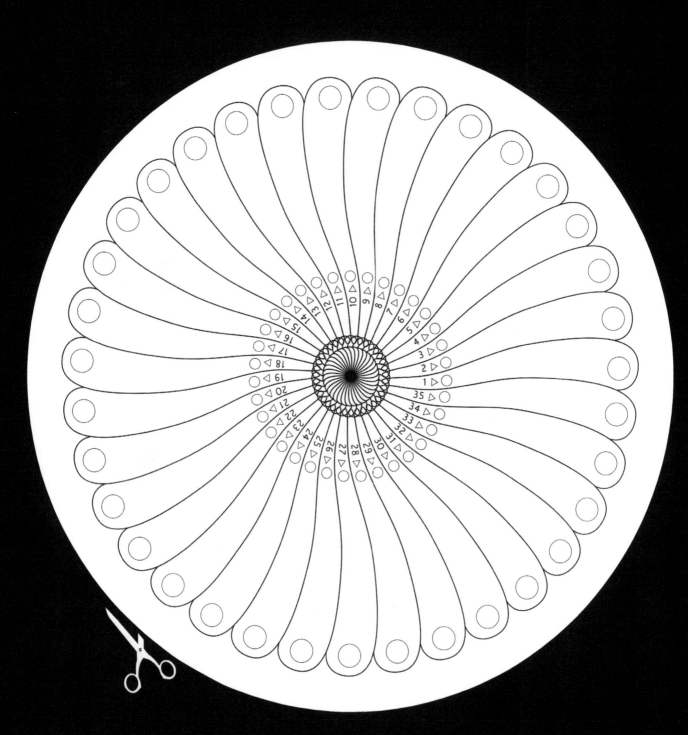

· PERSEPHONE ·

"I KNOW PAIN AND SADNESS; LIVING IN-BETWEEN WORLDS, I UNITE LIGHT AND DARKNESS; THE BOND WITH MY MOTHER SAVES ME."

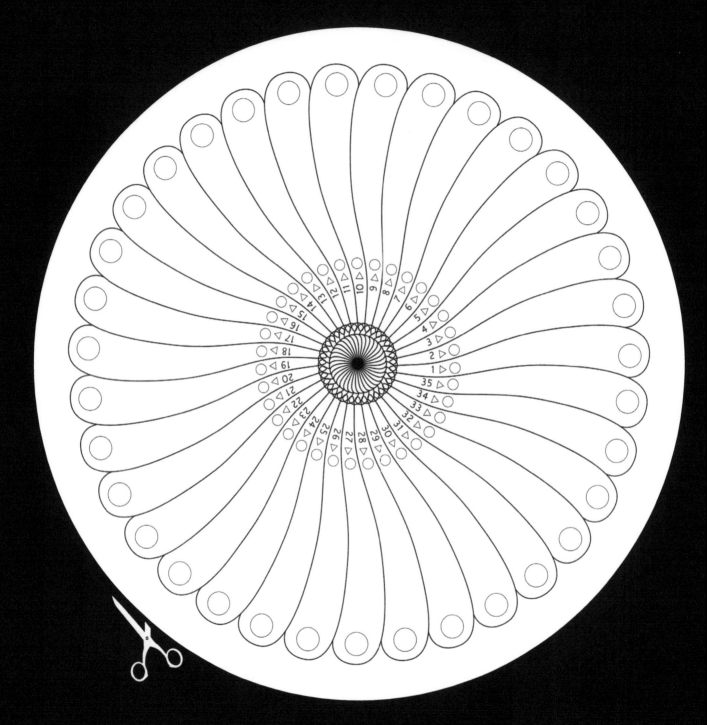

TISIPHONE

"I AM THE VOICE OF REVENGE AND I PUNISH THOSE WHO DO NOT RESPECT FAMILY TIES AND THE LIFE OF OTHERS."

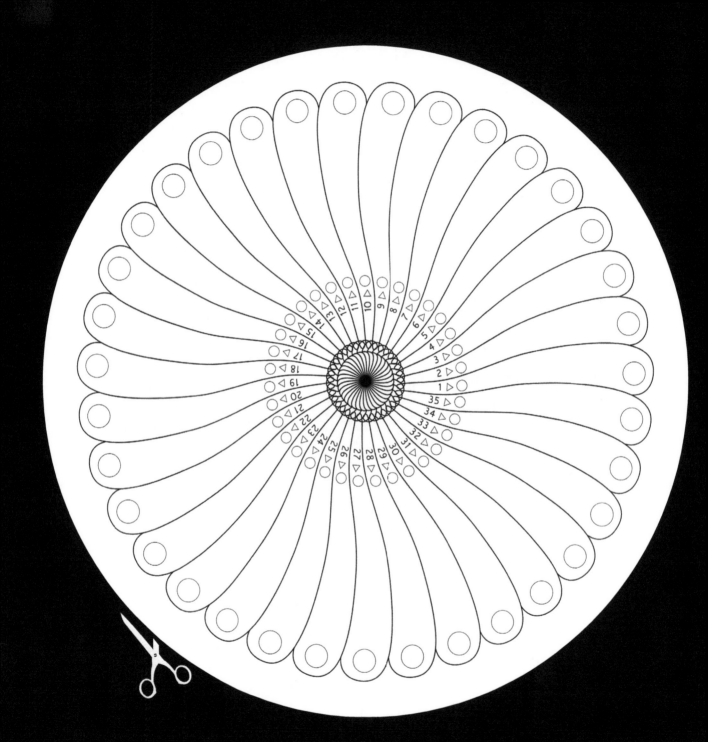

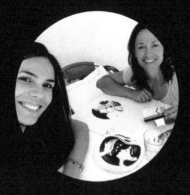

Care to send us your feedback or ideas?
We have a page for that:
facebook.com/thegoddessinyoubook/
See you soon! "

Who are we?

Ana and **Patrícia** first met in 2013 and share many passions. Ana draws, whilst Patrícia loves to talk.

They love to get together to talk about books and drawing, girls and moons, women and goddesses.

Patrícia's favourite goddess is Artemis – Ana even made them look alike! She finds that Demeter shows up whenever she's with her daughter, Antonia. She's also got something of Hestia and Alecto within her.

Ana awakes early to Aura, so that she can start her day on her bike or jogging in Nike and Artemis' company. While working, her pencil is guided by Tisiphone's warrior energies.

Together, Ana and Patrícia bring you this book so that you can discover who you truly are and learn to understand your body, taking good care of yourself, and others, cherishing and celebrating all the different sides of girlhood and womanhood.

You don't have to be like everybody else. You can just be you! Because you are – and you'll always be – a goddess in your own way.

"The Goddess in You" is especially created for girls aged 9-14 years, offering a unique, interactive approach to establishing cycle awareness, positive health and well-being.

It contains thirteen beautifully designed cycle mandalas, each illustrated with a goddess from Greek mythology.

Inspired by the archetypal work of the Jungian psychoanalysts, Clarissa Pinkola Estés and Jean Shinoda Bolen, *The Goddess in You* is a tool that works on many different levels. Through the charting of their menstrual cycle, girls will learn about their cyclical nature, internal rhythms and get a better understanding of their interaction with their own physical body. The goddess archetypes offer a diverse selection of female characteristics, to inspire self-awareness and self-acceptance, and celebrate the diversity of all the girls and women in each girl's life.

Easy to understand and attractive to use, this powerful book celebrates what it means to be a girl growing into womanhood.

Enjoy your cycles

Patrícia Lemos
Fertility Awareness Educator
circuloperfeito.com

Ana Afonso
Illustrator
anafonso.com

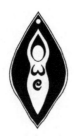

Womancraft
PUBLISHING

Life-changing, paradigm-shifting books
by women, for women

Visit us at: womancraftpublishing.com
Where you can sign up to the mailing list and receive samples of
our forthcoming titles before anyone else.

ⓕ WomancraftPublishing

ⓘ Womancraft_Publishing

Please leave a review of this book with your
favourite retalier or GoodReads.

Also from Womancraft

Reaching for the Moon: a girl's guide to her cycles

by Lucy H. Pearce

ISBN 978-1-910559-08-6

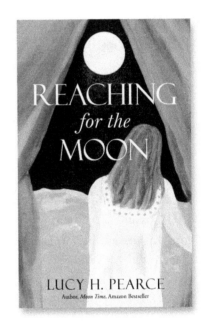

The girls' version of Lucy H. Pearce's Amazon bestselling book *Moon Time*. For girls aged 9-14, as they anticipate and experience their body's changes. *Reaching for the Moon* is a nurturing celebration of a girl's transformation to womanhood.

Beginning with an imaginary journey into the red tent, a traditional place of women's wisdom, gifts and secrets of womanhood are imparted in a gentle lyrical way. along with practical advice.

Now also available in the following translations:

Reiken naar de Maan (Dutch)
Rejoindre la Lune (French)
W Rytmie Księżyca (Polish)

A message of wonder, empowerment, magic and beauty in the shared secrets of our femininity ...written to encourage girls to embrace their transition to womanhood in a knowledgeable, supported, loving way.

thelovingparent.com

The Heroines Club: A Mother-Daughter Empowerment Circle

by Melia Keeton-Digby

ISBN 978-1-910559-14-7

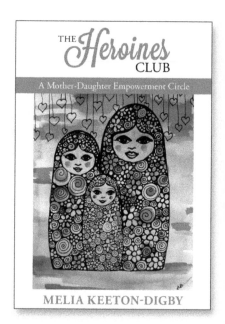

Nourishing guidance and a creative approach for mothers and daughters, aged 7+, to learn and grow together through the study of women's history. Each month focuses on a different heroine, featuring athletes, inventors, artists, and revolutionaries from around the world—including Frida Kahlo, Rosalind Franklin, Amelia Earhart, Anne Frank, Maya Angelou and Malala Yousafzai as strong role models for young girls to learn about, look up to, and be inspired by.

The Heroines Club is truly a must-have book for mothers who wish to foster a deeper connection with their daughters. As mothers, we are our daughter's first teacher, role model, and wise counsel. This book should be in every woman's hands, and passed down from generation to generation.
Wendy Cook, founder and facilitator of Mighty Girl Art

Lightning Source UK Ltd.
Milton Keynes UK
UKHW031916260122
397753UK00005B/180